Smoking

Pete Sanders and Steve Myers

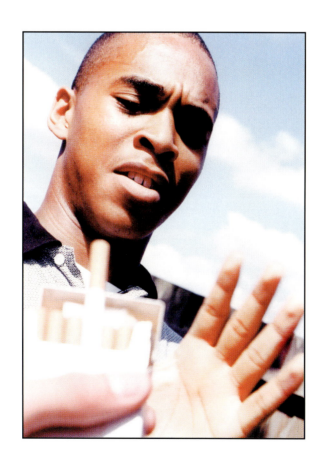

Aladdin / Watts
London • Sydney

© Aladdin Books Ltd 2004

Designed and produced by
Aladdin Books Ltd
28 Percy Street
London W1T 2BZ

New edition
first published in
Great Britain in 2004 by
Franklin Watts
96 Leonard Street
London EC2A 4XD

ISBN 0 7496 5493 7

Original edition published as
What Do You Know About –
Smoking

A catalogue record for this
book is available from the
British Library.

Printed in UAE
Editor
Harriet Brown

Designers
Flick, Book Design & Graphics
Simon Morse

Illustrator
Mike Lacey

Picture Research
Brian Hunter Smart

CONTENTS

Introduction   3

Why do people smoke?   4

Starting to smoke   7

What effect does smoking have
  on your health?   11

What other problems does
  smoking cause?   14

Passive smoking   18

The smoking industry   21

Stopping smoking   24

What can be done about smoking? 27

What can we do?   30

Useful addresses and websites   31

Index   32

How to use this book

The books in this series deal with issues that
affect the lives of many young people.
- Each book can be read by a young person
  alone, or together with an adult.
- Issues raised in the storyline are further
  discussed in accompanying text.
- Practical ideas are given in the 'What can
  we do?' section at the end of the book.
- Organisations and helplines are listed.

INTRODUCTION

" During our lifetime, we will all come into contact with smoking. You may have friends or family who smoke, or perhaps you know someone who is trying to give up. "

When Christopher Columbus returned from his discovery of the New World, he brought news of the strange custom of smoking rolled tobacco leaves. Tobacco has now been smoked in Europe in one form or another for hundreds of years. It was not until this century that cigarettes became fashionable. However, people's attitudes to smoking have changed a lot over the last few years.

Today, smoking raises many issues for adults and young people. You might be determined never to smoke, or you might be trying to decide whether to begin. This book will help you to understand more about the reasons why people smoke, the effects smoking has on health and ways of giving up smoking.

Each chapter focuses on a different aspect of the subject, illustrated by an episode in a continuing story. After each episode, we look at some of the issues raised, and widen out the discussion. By the end, you'll know more about all aspects of smoking, and will be able to make up your own mind about it.

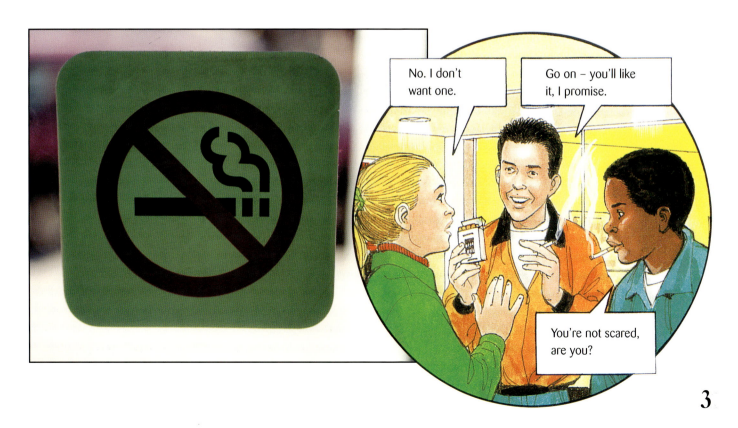

No. I don't want one.

Go on – you'll like it, I promise.

You're not scared, are you?

WHY DO PEOPLE SMOKE?

> Tobacco arrived in Europe in the 16th century. Many Europeans began to smoke because they believed tobacco contained medicine that would be good for their health.

Today, it is well-known that the opposite is true, and that smoking can be very dangerous. Yet many people, including young people, continue to smoke.

There are several reasons for this. Some smokers simply enjoy the taste of cigarettes. Or they feel smoking makes them look sophisticated. Some become used to the feel of a cigarette between their fingers, and find the act of taking a drag of a cigarette comforting. Some even claim cigarettes help them to think more clearly.

The main reason people smoke is that smoking quickly becomes a habit – an addiction. This is because cigarettes and other tobacco products contain a drug called nicotine. Nicotine is a deadly poison. The amount from cigarettes is not enough to kill, but it causes a serious reaction in the body. When tobacco smoke is inhaled, nicotine in the smoke passes into the bloodstream.

The drug reaches the brain in just a few seconds, making the smoker feel relaxed yet alert. Cigarettes also contain other chemicals, such as tar, ammonia and lead, which harm the body. Smoking can lead to cancer, heart disease and other health problems.

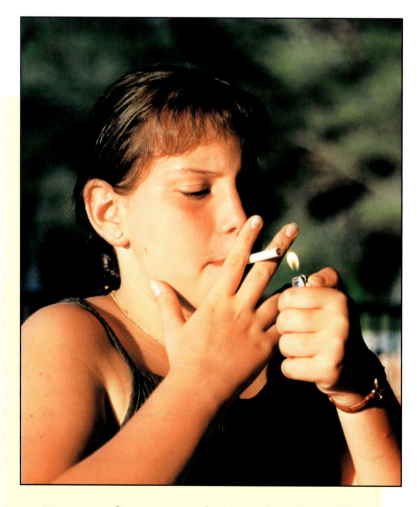

Once you have started to smoke, it can be very difficult to stop.

It was December...

... and Sarah and Sam Lawrence were shopping for presents with their mum, Barbara.

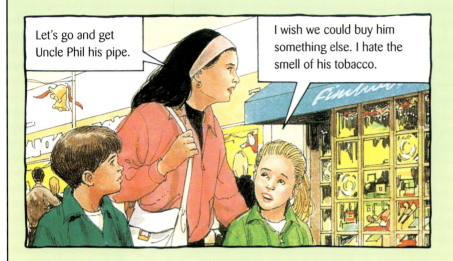

Let's go and get Uncle Phil his pipe.

I wish we could buy him something else. I hate the smell of his tobacco.

Whilst Mrs Lawrence paid for the pipe they had chosen, Sam and Sarah explored the shop.

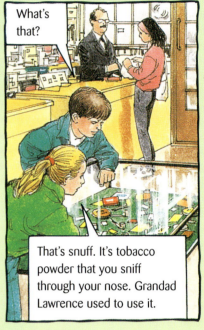

What's that?

That's snuff. It's tobacco powder that you sniff through your nose. Grandad Lawrence used to use it.

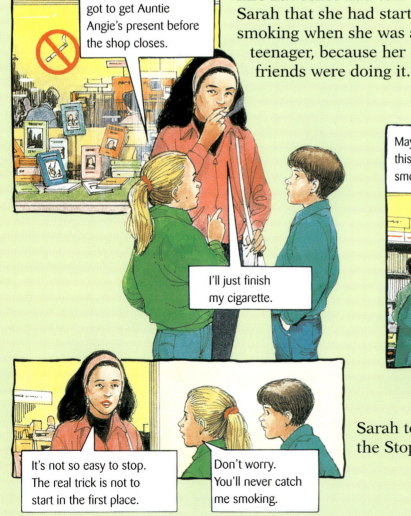

Come on, Mum. We've got to get Auntie Angie's present before the shop closes.

I'll just finish my cigarette.

Mrs Lawrence had told Sarah that she had started smoking when she was a teenager, because her friends were doing it.

It's not so easy to stop. The real trick is not to start in the first place.

Don't worry. You'll never catch me smoking.

Maybe we should get Mum this book on stopping smoking for Christmas.

I think she'd need more help than that. She's been smoking for years.

Sarah told her mum about the Stop Smoking book.

Do you think Sarah's mum is right?

5

That's snuff. It's tobacco powder that you sniff through your nose. Grandad Lawrence used to use it.

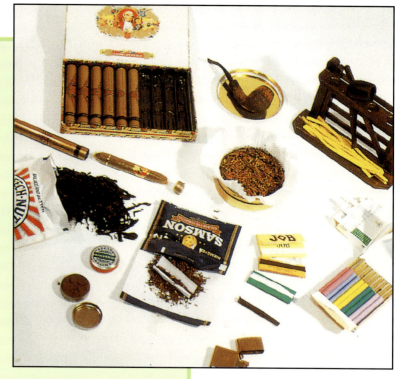

Cigarettes are the most popular tobacco product, and the most widely available. But tobacco is also available in other forms. Cigars and pipe-tobacco are lit and inhaled through the mouth, like cigarettes. Snuff is powdered tobacco which is sniffed or placed between the lip and gum. It was popular in the 18th century, but it's not used much today. Chewing tobacco is also sold. All these products contain nicotine.

I think she'd need more help than that. She's been smoking for years.

Sarah knows that her mum would find giving up smoking very hard, because she's smoked for years. Mrs Lawrence is addicted to nicotine. Her body has become so used to the drug that she would find it hard to do without it. Some people smoke as many as 60 cigarettes a day. 'Chain smokers' smoke one cigarette after another. They may light up a second cigarette without realising they haven't finished the first.

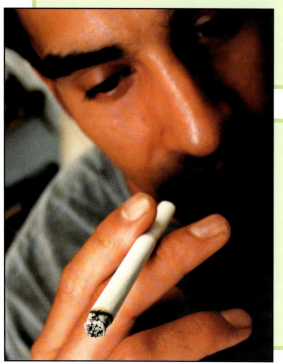

Like Mrs Lawrence, many parents do not want their children to smoke. Most adults are fully aware of the dangers involved in smoking, even if they cannot give up themselves, or feel they do not want to. As Mrs Lawrence knows, the only certain way not to let smoking become a problem is not to start in the first place.

STARTING TO SMOKE

" Two-thirds of all adults do not smoke. Most of those that do smoke start when they are young, usually in their early teens. "

Research suggests that if you have not started by the time you are 20 years old, it is likely that you will not become a smoker.

People start to smoke for different reasons. Older smokers may say they started because when they were younger, most of the people they knew smoked. In the past, people were less aware of the dangers involved, and there were no restrictions on advertising. Some adverts even made cigarettes appear to be good for you!

Some young people start to smoke because they say it makes them feel grown up. Some try cigarettes because they want to look big and impress others. Or they could be copying someone they admire, such as a celebrity. If your friends smoke, there is often a lot of pressure on you to take up smoking too. It can be hard to refuse when those around you are doing it. Whatever their reason for starting, people who take up smoking have not always considered the possible consequences later on.

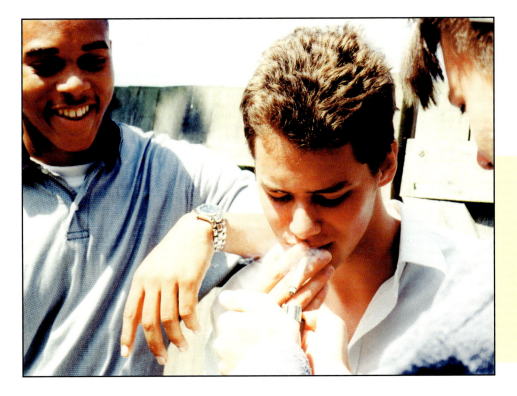

Some people begin to smoke simply because they have been told they mustn't. It is their way of rebelling; of showing they are different.

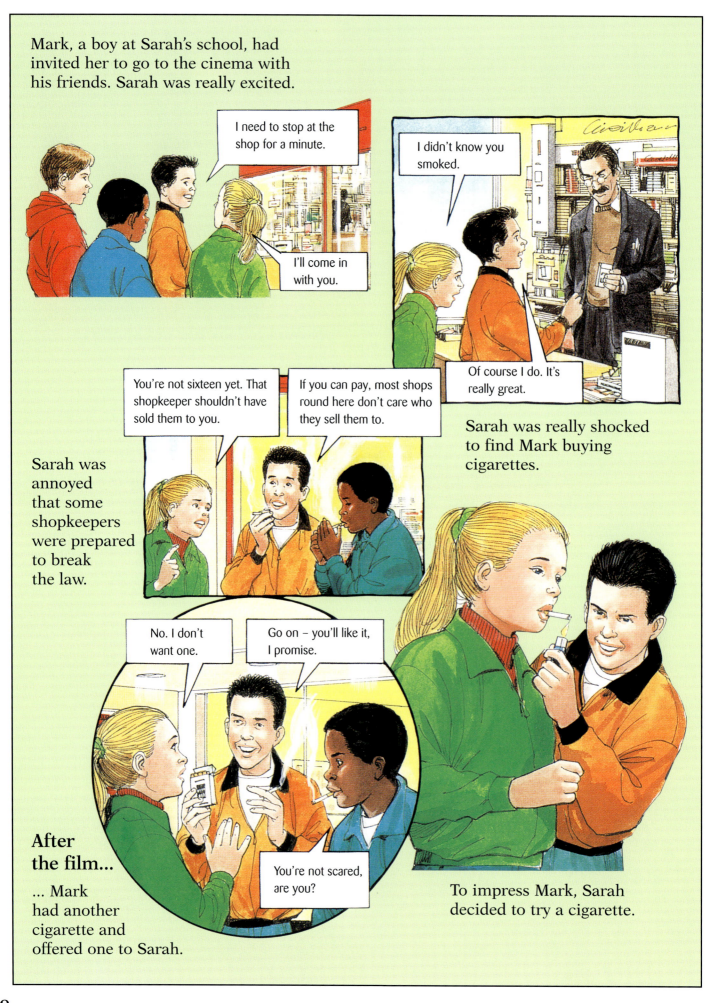

Mark, a boy at Sarah's school, had invited her to go to the cinema with his friends. Sarah was really excited.

I need to stop at the shop for a minute.

I'll come in with you.

I didn't know you smoked.

Of course I do. It's really great.

Sarah was really shocked to find Mark buying cigarettes.

You're not sixteen yet. That shopkeeper shouldn't have sold them to you.

If you can pay, most shops round here don't care who they sell them to.

Sarah was annoyed that some shopkeepers were prepared to break the law.

No. I don't want one.

Go on – you'll like it, I promise.

You're not scared, are you?

After the film...

... Mark had another cigarette and offered one to Sarah.

To impress Mark, Sarah decided to try a cigarette.

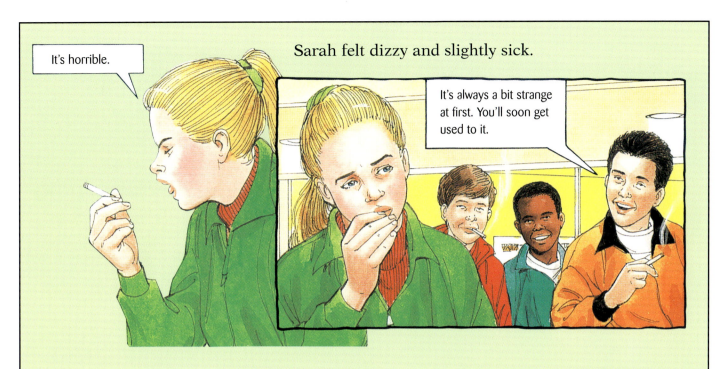

Sarah felt dizzy and slightly sick.

It's horrible.

It's always a bit strange at first. You'll soon get used to it.

Christmas Day

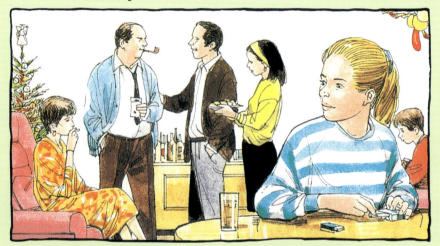

Mark was right. By Christmas, Sarah had grown to like cigarettes, and had begun to steal her mum's.

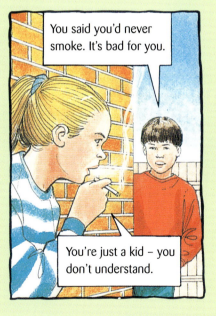

You said you'd never smoke. It's bad for you.

You're just a kid – you don't understand.

Sam noticed Sarah sneak out of the house, and followed her.

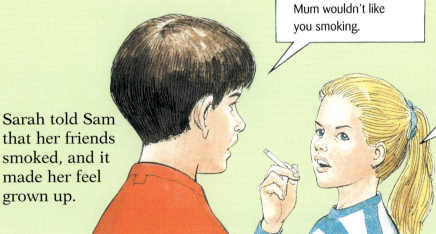

Mum wouldn't like you smoking.

I can give up any time I want to. And you'd better not tell anyone about this.

Sarah told Sam that her friends smoked, and it made her feel grown up.

9

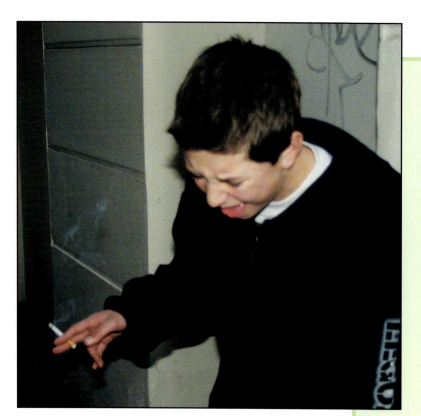

It's always a bit strange at first. You'll soon get used to it.

The reaction to the first cigarette varies from person to person. Some people find it makes them feel slightly dizzy. Others feel sick. Nicotine causes all these effects, which are symptoms of very mild poisoning. Sarah did not enjoy her first cigarette very much, but Mark persuaded her to keep trying. She got used to the taste – and to the feeling she got from smoking. Addiction happens very quickly.

There are laws about the age at which you can buy cigarettes.

However, many shops are prepared to break the law.

- Young people who are determined to smoke will find ways to get hold of cigarettes.

- If a shop refuses to serve them, they may ask someone older to buy them on their behalf.

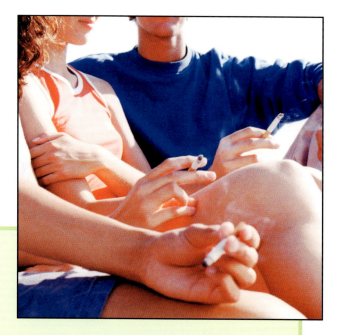

Go on – you'll like it, I promise. You're not scared are you?

Surveys carried out in Britain have shown that people often start smoking at the age of 11 or 12, at the time when they change schools. This can be a particularly difficult time for many young people. If you are trying to make new friends, it can be hard to refuse to do what they are doing – even if you know it is wrong. You want to be accepted. But remember that real friends will not try to force you to do things you don't want to do.

WHAT EFFECT DOES SMOKING HAVE ON YOUR HEALTH?

> " Worldwide, about four million people die prematurely each year as a result of smoking. "

The smoke from burning tobacco contains more than 4,000 gases and chemicals, many of which are poisonous. These substances include ammonia, found in cleaning fluids, carbon monoxide, the deadly gas in car exhaust fumes, and tar. When cigarette smoke is inhaled, these substances pass into the body.

A smoker breathes cigarette smoke directly through the mouth into the bronchial tubes which lead to the lungs. Tiny particles stick to the walls of the tubes, causing irritation. The cigarette smoke which passes into the lungs leaves behind a sticky brown tar. This tar contains chemicals known to cause cancer. Nine out of ten deaths from lung cancer are caused by smoking.

Smoking can lead to cancer of the mouth and throat. It can cause other breathing problems. The body produces mucus to try to protect itself from the effects of tar. This can sometimes clog the air passages and the lungs, and they can no longer work properly. This can be fatal. Smokers also run the risk of developing heart disease. Because of the effects of nicotine and carbon monoxide on the blood, the heart has to work harder to get the oxygen it needs. Smoking also increases the amount of fatty deposits in the arteries. This can lead to a heart attack. Smokers are twice as likely to have a heart attack than non-smokers.

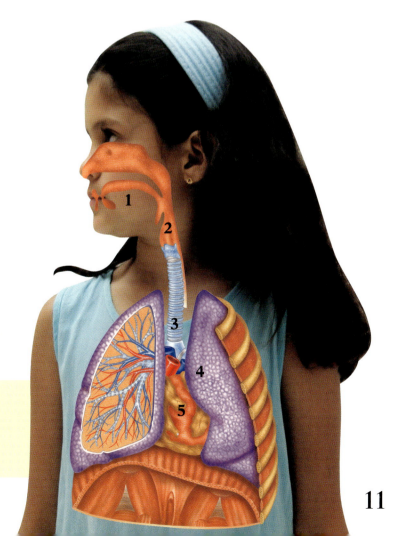

Smoking can damage the mouth (1), throat (2), bronchial tubes (3), lungs (4) and heart (5).

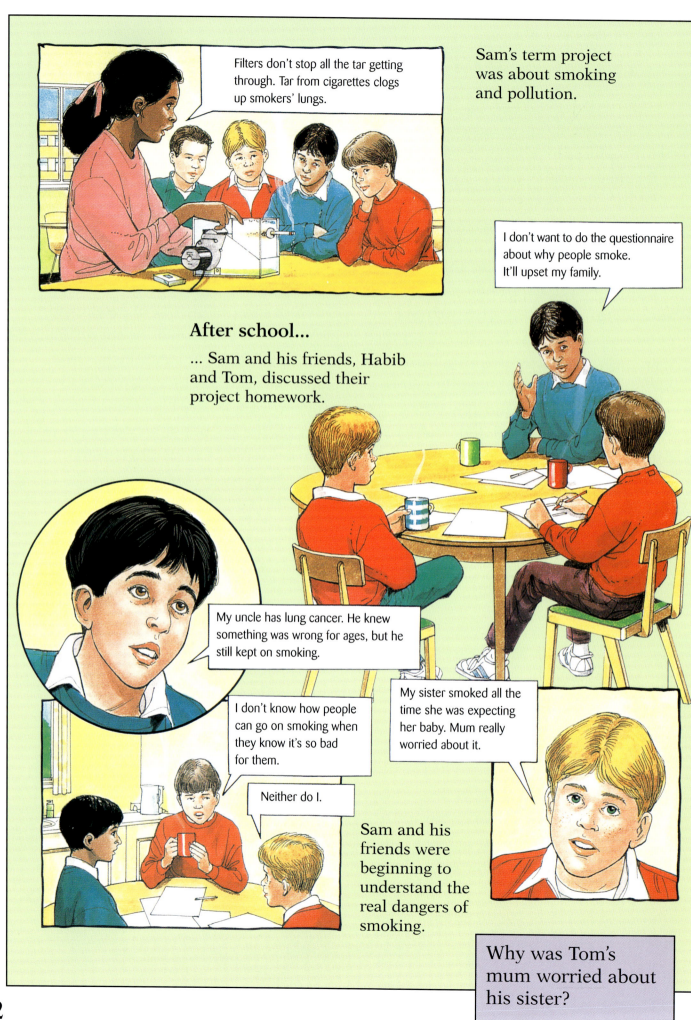

Filters don't stop all the tar getting through. Tar from cigarettes clogs up smokers' lungs.

Sam's term project was about smoking and pollution.

I don't want to do the questionnaire about why people smoke. It'll upset my family.

After school...

... Sam and his friends, Habib and Tom, discussed their project homework.

My uncle has lung cancer. He knew something was wrong for ages, but he still kept on smoking.

My sister smoked all the time she was expecting her baby. Mum really worried about it.

I don't know how people can go on smoking when they know it's so bad for them.

Neither do I.

Sam and his friends were beginning to understand the real dangers of smoking.

Why was Tom's mum worried about his sister?

12

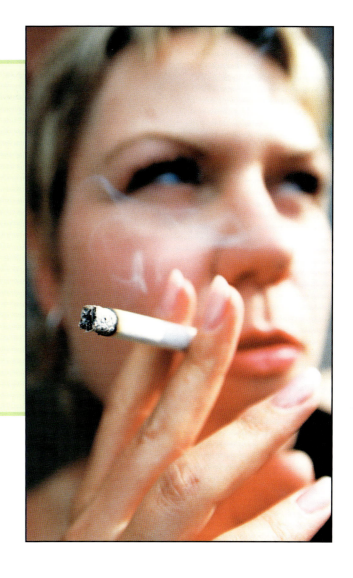

> My sister smoked all the time she was expecting her baby. Mum really worried about it.

Tom is aware that his sister took a big risk by smoking when she was pregnant.
If a woman smokes while she is pregnant, chemicals from the smoke enter her bloodstream and also the bloodstream of her unborn child. Research has shown that pregnant women who smoke stand a higher risk of their baby dying than those who don't. There's also a greater chance that babies will be born prematurely, or will not weigh as much as they should.

> He knew something was wrong for ages, but he still kept on smoking.

Habib's uncle thought that smoking wouldn't harm him.
Smokers are tempted to think 'it won't happen to me'. They might tell you about people who have smoked all their lives and lived to a very old age. For some people this is the case, but it does not mean that smoking hasn't affected their health. People die every day from diseases that are directly caused by smoking.

Sam's teacher has helped the class to understand that the long-term effects of smoking are devastating.
Sometimes smokers themselves are not aware that the diseases caused by smoking usually occur gradually, after someone has been smoking for many years. Because they feel fine, smokers may be ignoring the fact that they are running a large risk of serious illness at some point later in life.

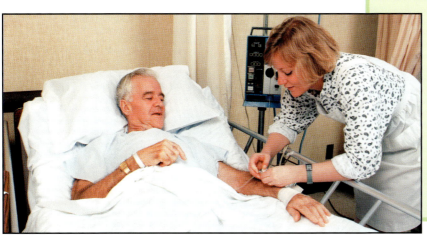

WHAT OTHER PROBLEMS DOES SMOKING CAUSE?

 It is said that the tobacco industry needs 300 new smokers each day, just to replace those who have died.

The risk of major illness caused by smoking is well known. However, apart from the health hazards, smoking can also lead to less obvious problems.

Smokers may find that they enjoy food less because cigarettes can affect the way you taste food. Tar and nicotine deposits can build up on the teeth, making them discoloured. A smoker's fingers may be stained yellow from holding cigarettes. A great many smokers complain of 'smoker's cough'. This is the body's way of trying to get rid of some of the tar that has settled in the bronchial tubes, by producing extra mucus to clear the lungs. It is usually worst in the mornings, when the smoker has just woken up.

Smoking also makes people less fit. Many smokers get out of breath very easily, and take longer to recover from any form of exercise than non-smokers. These symptoms can signal the beginnings of serious health problems. Often, however, smokers choose to ignore the symptoms, or do not realise how great the risks are. They may continue to smoke and suffer from serious illness later in life.

Your ability to play and enjoy sport could be damaged by smoking.

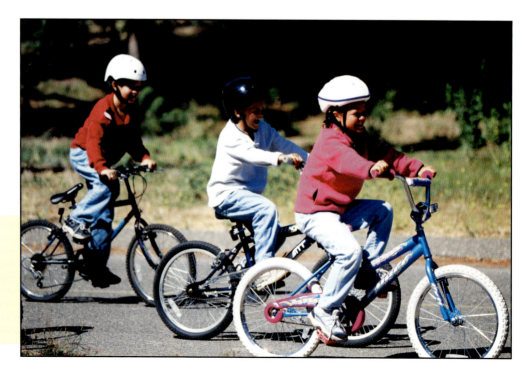

As part of the project, Sam's class had to design posters about smoking.

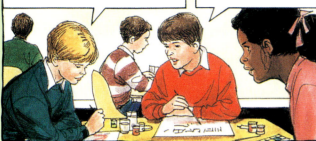

Sam was pleased with his poster and asked to take it home.

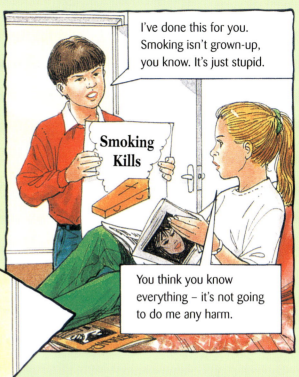

Sam told Sarah that he had learnt in class that smoking now can cause serious illnesses later on.

Sarah refused to listen. She tore up Sam's poster and stormed out.

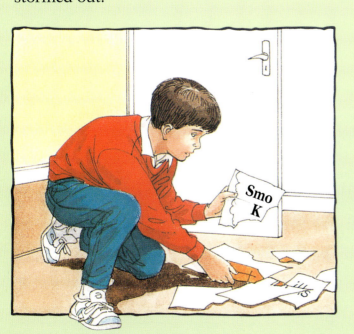

Nobody seemed very happy that evening. Sarah and Sam weren't talking to each other, and their dad was also annoyed.

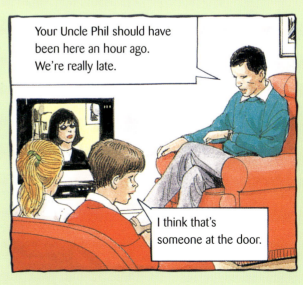

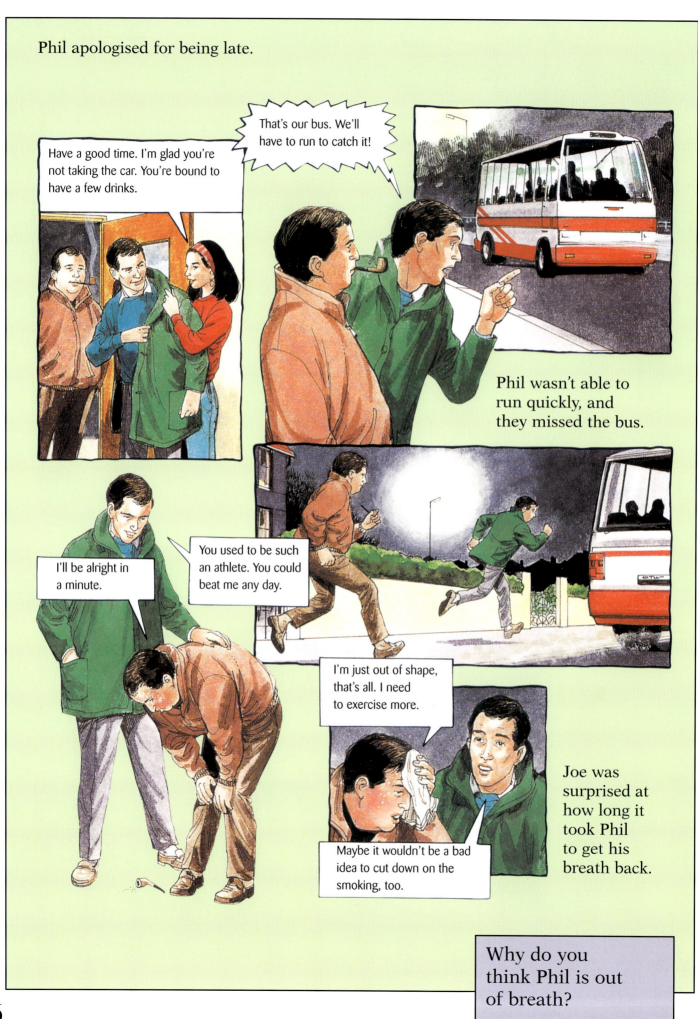

Phil apologised for being late.

That's our bus. We'll have to run to catch it!

Have a good time. I'm glad you're not taking the car. You're bound to have a few drinks.

Phil wasn't able to run quickly, and they missed the bus.

I'll be alright in a minute.

You used to be such an athlete. You could beat me any day.

I'm just out of shape, that's all. I need to exercise more.

Maybe it wouldn't be a bad idea to cut down on the smoking, too.

Joe was surprised at how long it took Phil to get his breath back.

Why do you think Phil is out of breath?

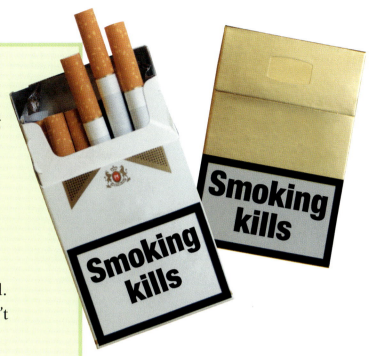

You used to be such an athlete. You could beat me any day. Maybe you should cut down your smoking.

All tobacco products carry a warning about the health hazards involved in smoking. But the message isn't getting through as well as it should. Phil was an athlete, but now finds it difficult to run even a short distance. This is because his lungs have been damaged by smoking over a long period. However, this kind of warning often isn't enough to alter people's behaviour.

Mine's about fire. Loads of fires are caused by people not putting out cigarettes properly.

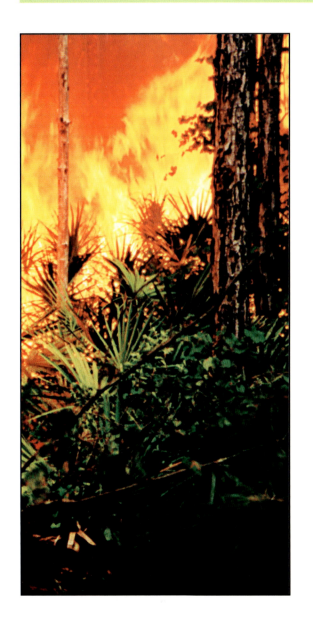

As Tom and Sam know, the other great risk from smoking is fire. A great many fires are caused by cigarettes or matches not being put out properly. Many people have been killed because they have fallen asleep in bed with a lighted cigarette, and set fire to bedclothes. Many places have banned smoking completely because of the risk of fire.

Forest fires
In some parts of the world, huge areas of land have been destroyed by forest fires.

• Often these fires have been started by just one cigarette or match thrown away carelessly.

• Fires quickly take hold and get out of control. Trees, plants, animals and even humans die.

PASSIVE SMOKING

"Research has proved that smokers are not only putting their own health at risk by smoking."

'Passive smoking' – breathing in the smoke coming from other people's cigarettes – greatly increases our chances of developing serious health problems, even if we are not smokers ourselves.

If you have ever walked into a room where lots of people are smoking, you will have noticed smoke filling the air. Smoke can get into people's hair and clothes, and make them smell unpleasant.

Passive smoking can make you cough, or give you a sore throat, a runny nose or a headache. It can be particularly harmful to people who suffer from asthma. Scientists have now shown that passive smokers also run the risk of developing the same kinds of major diseases as regular smokers. For this reason, more and more people are calling for a ban on smoking in all public venues. This has already happened in some parts of the world, such as California, USA.

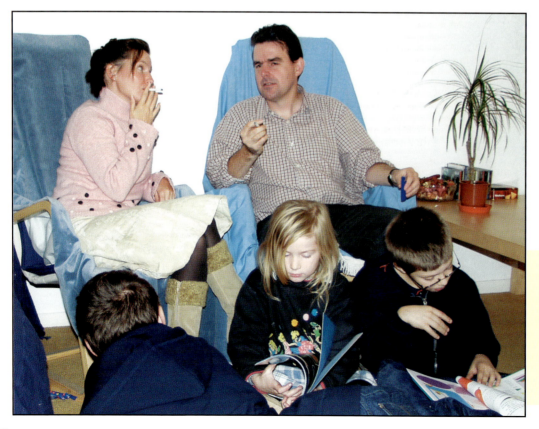

Breathing other people's cigarette smoke can be as bad for you as smoking yourself.

It was April 21st...

... which was Mark's birthday. He had invited Sarah to join in the family party.

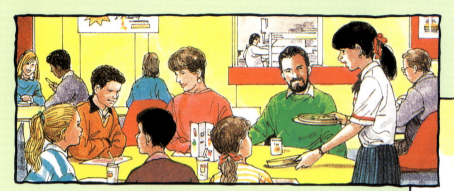

After he had finished his meal, Mark's father lit a cigarette.

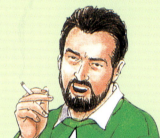

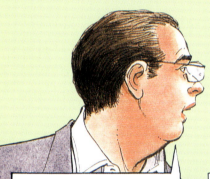

Excuse me. Would you mind putting your cigarette out?

Yes, I would, as a matter of fact.

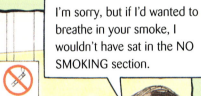

I'm sorry, but if I'd wanted to breathe in your smoke, I wouldn't have sat in the NO SMOKING section.

I can remember a time when you could smoke when and where you wanted to. Nobody bothered you.

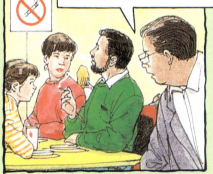

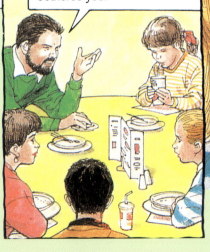

Actually, smoking's okay, but I still don't like people smoking when I'm eating.

Realising he was in the wrong, Mark's father put out his cigarette.

Should all restaurants ban smoking altogether?

19

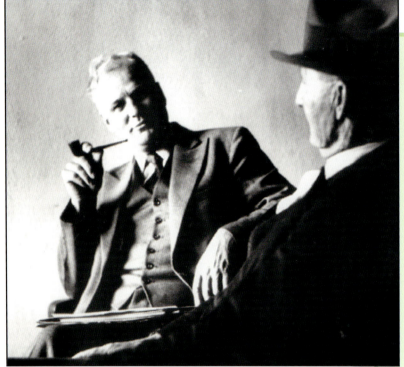

Non-smoking areas

Most forms of public transport, shops and cinemas have banned smoking altogether.

- Restaurants often have smoking and non-smoking areas. But, although the restaurant can say where smokers should sit, it has little control over the smoke.

- Smoking is banned in some open-air parks, particularly in California, USA.

Many people have strong opinions about smoking.

It is said that smokers have the right to choose to smoke. However, anti-smoking organisations call for a complete ban on smoking in public places and offices. They say that smokers should not have the right to put other people's health at risk through passive smoking.

I remember a time when you could smoke when and where you wanted to. Nobody bothered you.

People's views about smoking have changed a great deal over the years.

Mark's father remembers a time when nobody minded if you smoked. Smoking was seen to be fashionable. Films and advertising companies encouraged people, particularly women, to take up smoking. They always showed smokers having a good time, and gave the impression that smoking made people attractive. One cigarette company even used doctors to advertise its cigarettes.

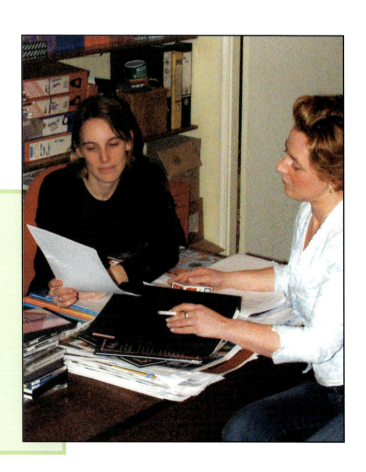

THE SMOKING INDUSTRY

" Smoking is big business. Every year, tobacco companies earn billions of pounds from the sale of their products. They spend millions on advertising, to encourage more people to buy. "

Tobacco is grown in most parts of the world. Tobacco companies pay farmers to grow the crop. In many cases, the farmers can make more money from growing tobacco than from growing food.

In some developing countries this has had serious consequences. Much-needed food crops are not planted, because the land is being used to grow tobacco. Tobacco farmers also use a lot of pesticides to make sure the harvest is large. Pesticides can get into drinking water, drift onto food crops and harm animals.

In recent years, the hazards of smoking have become clear. Governments have forced cigarette companies to print a large health warning on every packet. Tobacco companies started to produce different 'strengths' of cigarettes, containing high, middle or low amounts of tar. Sales of high tar brands have fallen in countries where people are aware of the dangers. Yet these brands are still popular in the developing world where health education is not as effective. However, there is debate over whether smoking 'low tar' cigarettes is any better for your health than smoking 'normal' cigarettes.

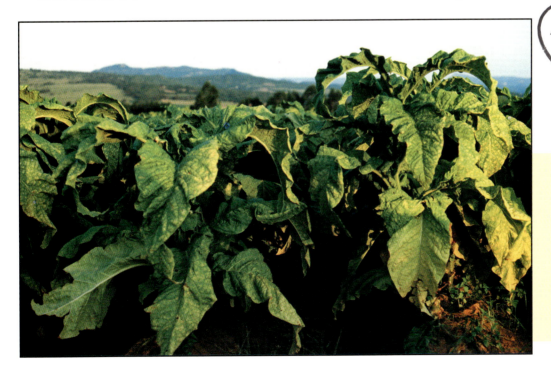

Tobacco uses up the goodness from the soil, making it less fertile for other crops.

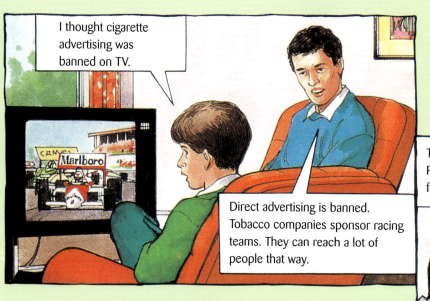

Sam was watching sport on the TV with his dad. He was surprised to see cigarette brands advertised on racing cars.

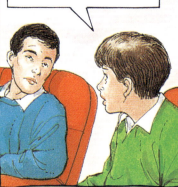

Joe told Barbara what Sam had said. They decided to confront Sarah.

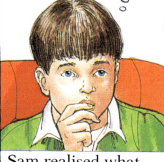

Sam realised what he had said.

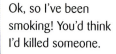

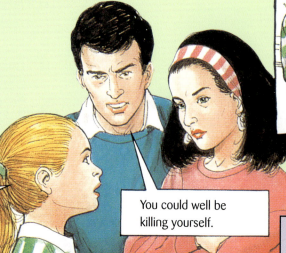

When things had cooled down Barbara talked to Sarah again.

Should all cigarette adverts be banned all over the world?

22

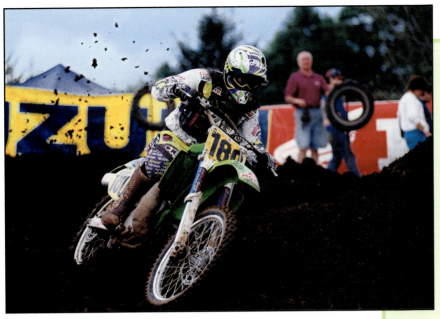

Tobacco companies sponsor racing teams. They can reach a lot of people that way.

Governments of many countries have banned direct advertising of cigarettes on television. Some tobacco companies sponsor racing teams, for example. This means that when TV programmes show these events, the name of the company will be shown or mentioned. In countries that have banned tobacco advertising, the adverts must be removed from the cars. There are plans for a global ban on cigarette advertising.

All over the world, governments make a lot of money from taxes on cigarettes. In the UK, over three-quarters of the price of a packet of cigarettes is tax, which goes to the government. The amounts involved are so great that governments have come to rely on the money they receive. Yet governments could save a great deal on health care. It costs millions every year to look after people who are ill from smoking-related diseases.

All tobacco advertising should be banned. It makes smoking look cool. That's why Sarah started.

Governments in some countries no longer allow cigarette adverts to link smoking with success and health. To overcome this, posters advertising cigarettes have become more unusual. Companies have found ways of suggesting a brand just by using a certain colour. In the UK, even this type of advertising has now been banned. Tobacco companies are likely to invest in advertising in countries with fewer restrictions on tobacco advertising.

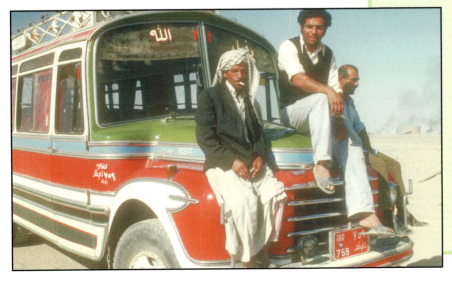

STOPPING SMOKING

Many smokers would like to stop. But the habit of smoking can be hard to break. It does not help to blame smokers for being addicted.

Most people agree that to be successful, a person must really want to stop. Smokers must make the decision for themselves.

Smokers often have mistaken ideas about what will happen if they stop. Some assume they'll get fat. If they replace cigarettes with snacks, they will put on weight. But stopping smoking itself does not make you fat. Some people gradually cut down the number of cigarettes they smoke. Others stop smoking altogether straight away. Hypnosis and acupuncture are sometimes used to take away the urge to smoke. Special products can help smokers give up. Nicotine chewing gum, and patches which are attached to the skin like a plaster, help reduce the craving for cigarettes, by giving a temporary boost of nicotine. Often it can help to get professional help to give up smoking. Some helplines are listed at the end of this book. Some people consider how much money they will save by quitting and others ask for help and motivation from friends and family.

Taking the decision to stop can be as hard as stopping itself.

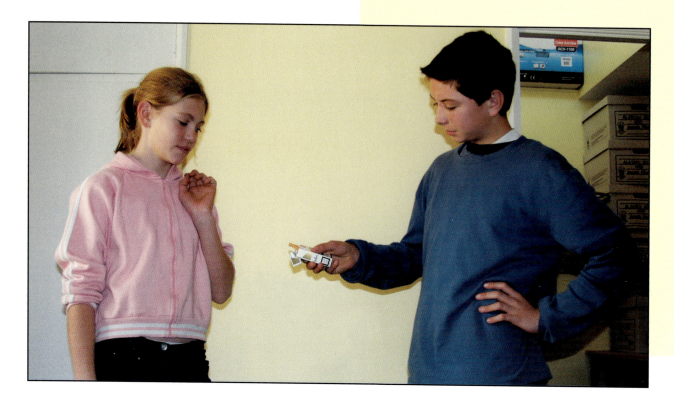

A month after Sarah and Barbara had stopped smoking...

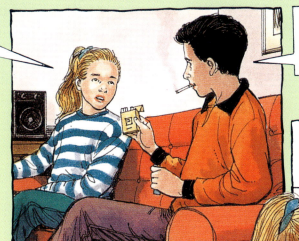

You know I've given up. So has Mum.

Everyone's out – they'll never know. Come on, have one. It won't do you any harm.

It DOES do you harm. For one thing, it makes your breath smell – not to mention what it does to your insides.

Later...

... Sarah talked to her mum.

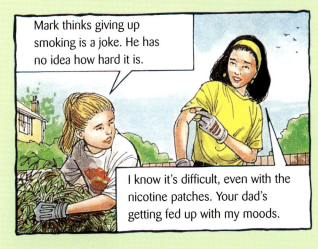

Mark thinks giving up smoking is a joke. He has no idea how hard it is.

I know it's difficult, even with the nicotine patches. Your dad's getting fed up with my moods.

Sarah was annoyed with Mark for trying to persuade her to smoke again.

A week later...

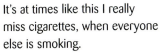

... Barbara was having lunch with Phil's wife, Angie.

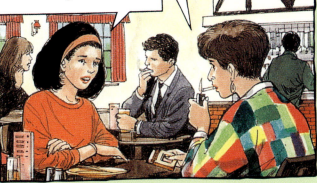

It's at times like this I really miss cigarettes, when everyone else is smoking.

Well help yourself to one of mine if you really want one.

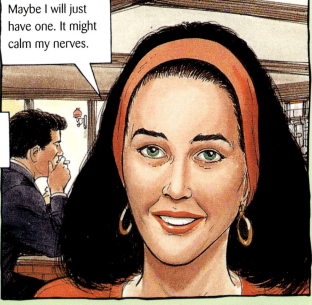

Maybe I will just have one. It might calm my nerves.

Did Angie help by offering Barbara a cigarette?

For one thing, it makes your breath smell.

Sarah now feels that smoking is not an attractive habit.
The smell of cigarette smoke lingers in people's clothes and in their hair. Smokers may also find that cigarettes make their breath smell. Non-smokers are often put off by these things.

Cravings
Stopping smoking deprives the body of the nicotine it is used to.

- People may become moody and irritable as their bodies slowly try to adjust to this change.

- They may be stressed and easily upset. The moods are the fault of the nicotine, not the person.

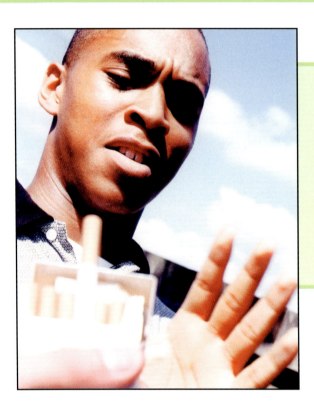

Angie made it harder for Barbara to give up smoking, by offering her a cigarette.
Many smokers find the hardest part of giving up is being in social situations. Often when people around them are smoking, the desire to smoke can be very strong indeed.

Maybe I will just have one. It might calm my nerves.

Like Barbara, some former smokers do go back to smoking.
They may explain this by saying they were under great stress, lacked willpower or were feeling fed-up. Smoking becomes such a part of people's lives that they need help from friends and family in order to stop.

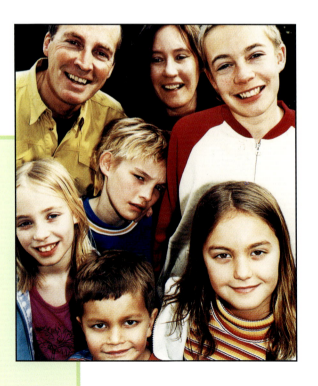

WHAT CAN BE DONE ABOUT SMOKING?

A survey found that a quarter of those asked had tried their first cigarette before the age of ten.

For the tobacco industry, every young person addicted to smoking means years of profit. A full understanding of the facts about smoking might help us to decide it's best never to start.

If the health hazards involved in smoking are so bad, why don't governments ban smoking altogether? The truth is that governments make a great deal of money from taxing cigarettes. A government that banned smoking completely would face pressure from the tobacco industry, and would be accused of taking away people's right to choose. It would lose the votes of many smokers, and would be unlikely to be re-elected.

It has been suggested that cigarettes should be made even more expensive. But putting up the price of a product which is addictive may not discourage people from buying it. Certainly, there should be tougher action taken against shopkeepers who sell cigarettes to young people. Some organisations call for even more places to be made into non-smoking areas, including outdoor public places such as parks.

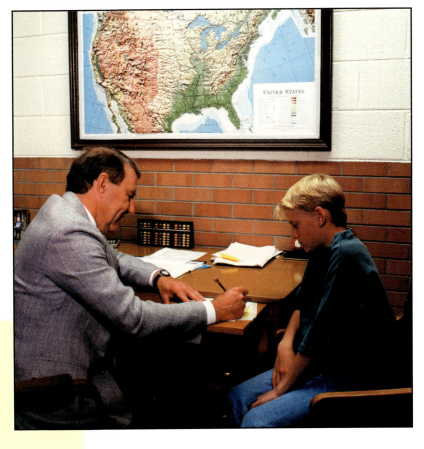

Perhaps everyone should be given information about the problems and dangers of smoking at an early age.

Barbara began to smoke regularly again.
But the family persuaded her to have
another try at stopping.

Sarah had heard her
mum and dad talking.

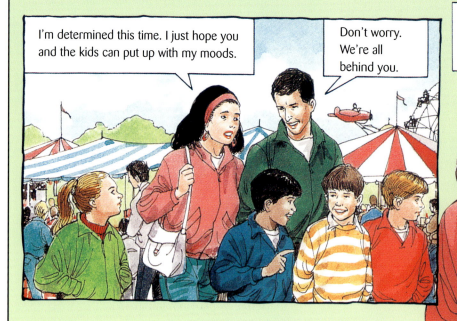

I'm determined this time. I just hope you and the kids can put up with my moods.

Don't worry. We're all behind you.

I think you should put the money you save by not smoking into a special bank account.

Good idea. Cigarettes are so expensive, you'd soon have a small fortune to spend on yourself.

Later...

... Sarah ran into Mark.

I'm thinking of stopping myself. People have told me I smell like an ashtray.

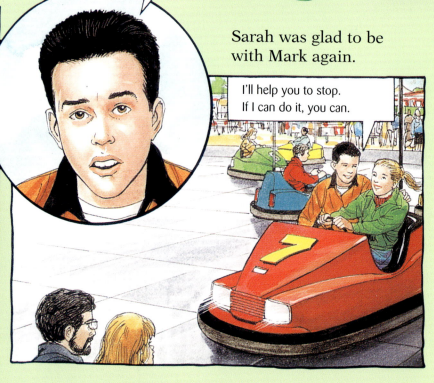

I'm sorry I gave you a hard time about not smoking.

Sarah was glad to be with Mark again.

I'll help you to stop. If I can do it, you can.

I tried to blame you, but it was my decision to start in the first place.

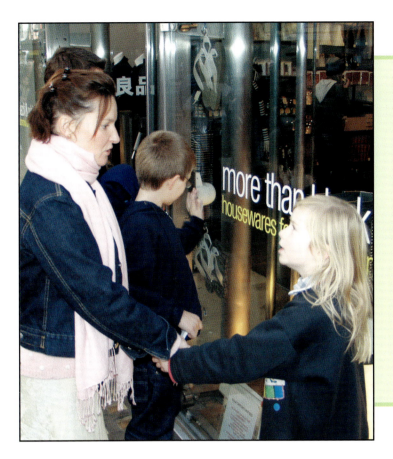

Sarah's idea of putting money away is helping her mum to stop smoking. Cigarettes are expensive, so the money saved through not smoking can build up quickly. People see their savings grow each week and know that this is money which would otherwise literally have been burned. In rewarding themselves from time to time by buying something special, they are strengthening their decision not to smoke any more. They start to look forward to the next 'reward'.

> I'll help you to stop. If I can do it, you can.

> I'm determined this time. I just hope you and the kids can put up with my moods.

People who are trying to give up need a lot of support from those around them. Some smokers have found that giving up at the same time as others who want to stop can help. Anyone who is having difficulty can discuss the problem with people who are in the same situation, who understand how they are feeling. There are also many organisations dedicated to helping people give up smoking. Some are listed on page 31.

Barbara, Sarah and Mark are going to have to work hard not to smoke in the future. Barbara is determined not to start smoking again. No Smoking Days have helped some addicted smokers like her to

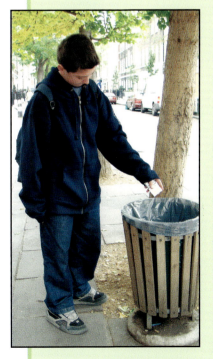

take the decision to give up. Sarah is annoyed that she started to smoke at all. She understands that she had the right to refuse the cigarettes Mark offered her. She chose to accept because she wanted to impress him. Mark now feels he was wrong to persuade her to start.

WHAT CAN WE DO?

" Having read this book, you will understand more about why people smoke, and the effect smoking can have on our lives. "

If you have thought about taking up smoking, or have tried it already, you need to consider the damage it can do to your health.

Remember, smoking is not glamorous. You only have to look at an ashtray full of cigarette ends to see that. If you do smoke, don't offer cigarettes to your friends. By encouraging others to smoke, you are putting them at risk too. You can reduce the amount of tar and nicotine you take into your body by taking fewer puffs or smoking less of each cigarette. This still does not make cigarettes safe, though. Some smokers find giving up tobacco difficult; others don't. As soon as you give up, the health risks begin to decrease and you can start living a healthier life.

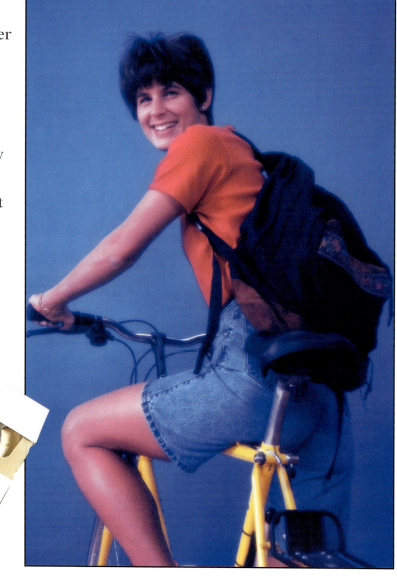

Smoking affects everyone – not just the people who are smoking. Adults can help by understanding that young people are often copying them when they smoke. The children of smokers are more likely to take up the habit than the children of non-smokers.

Anyone trying to quit may be able to get support or advice from some of the organisations listed below. If you know someone who has stopped, help them by giving encouragement and praise. It can be difficult to quit but it can be done.

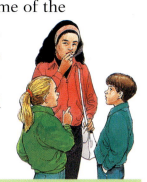

ASH (Action on Smoking and Health) England
(ASH is a public health charity dedicated to the reduction and eventual elimination of the health problems caused by tobacco.)
102 Clifton Street
London
EC2A 4HW
Tel: +44 (0) 207 739 5902
Email: enquiries@ash.org.uk
Website: www.ash.org.uk

ASH (Action on Smoking and Health) Scotland
8 Frederick Street
Edinburgh
EH2 2HB
Scotland
Tel: +44 (0) 131 225 4725
Email: ashscotland@ashscotland.org.uk
Website: www.ashscotland.org.uk

British Heart Foundation
14 Fitzhardinge Street
London
W1H 6DH
Tel: +44 (0) 207 935 0185
Helpline: 08450 70 80 70
(Mon-Fri 9am-5pm)
Email: internet@bhf.org.uk
Website: www.bhf.org.uk

Cancer Research Campaign
PO Box 123
Lincoln's Inn Fields
London
WC2A 3PX
Tel: +44 (0) 207 009 8820
Website: www.crc.org.uk

QUIT
Ground Floor
211 Old Street
London
EC1V 9NR
Quitline: 0800 00 22 00
Email: stopsmoking@quit.org.uk
Website: www.quit.org.uk

The Teacher's Advisory Council on Alcohol and Drugs Education
Old Exchange Building
St Ann's Passage
Manchester M2 6AF
Tel: +44 (0) 161 836 6850
Email: info@tacade.com
Website: www.tacade.com

Ulster Cancer Foundation
40-42 Eglantine Avenue
Belfast
BT9 6DX
Northern Ireland
Tel: +44 (0) 28 9066 3281
Email: info@ulstercancer.org
Website: www.ulstercancer.org

ASH (Action on Smoking and Health) New Zealand
Level 2
27 Gillies Avenue
PO Box 99-126
Newmarket
Auckland
New Zealand
Tel: +64 (0) 9 520 4866
Email: ashnz@ash.org.nz
Website: www.ash.org.nz

Canadian Cancer Society
(Look under 'Risk Reduction' for lots of information on tobacco and smoking, its effects on health and ways of giving up.)
National Office
Suite 200
10 Alcorn Avenue
Toronto
Ontario
M4V 3B1
Tel: +1 (0) 416 961 7223
Email: ccs@cancer.ca
Website: www.cancer.ca

The Australian Council on Smoking and Health
Level 1
46 Ventnor Avenue
West Perth, 6005
Western Australia
Tel: +61 (0) 8 9212 4300
Email: info@acosh.org
Website: www.acosh.org

INDEX

A
addiction 4, 6, 10, 24
advertising 7, 20, 21, 22, 23, 27
asthma 18
attitudes to smoking 20

B
bans on smoking 18, 20, 27
breathing problems 11, 16, 18

C
cancer 4, 11, 13, 31
chain smokers 6
chemicals in smoke 4, 11, 13
children of smokers 31
cigarette smoke 4, 11
cigars and pipe tobacco 6
cravings 26

F
fire, risk of 15, 17
first cigarette 8, 9, 10, 27

fitness, lack of 14, 16, 17

G
government action 23, 27

H
health care costs 23
health hazards and other problems 4, 11, 12, 13, 14, 17, 18, 21, 27, 30
heart disease 4, 11
history 4, 6

L
laws about selling cigarettes 9, 10

N
nicotine 4, 6, 10, 11, 13, 14, 24, 26, 30
non-smoking areas 20, 27

O
organisations that can help 29, 30-1

P
passive smoking 18, 20
pipe tobacco 5, 6
pregnancy, smoking during 12, 13

R
reasons for smoking 4, 7
restaurant, smoking in 20

S
saving money 28, 29
smoker's cough 14
snuff 5, 6
social situations 26
sponsorship 22, 23
starting smoking 5, 7, 8, 9, 10
stopping smoking 4, 5, 22, 24, 25, 26, 29, 30, 31

T
tar 4, 11, 12, 14, 21, 30
tax on cigarettes 23, 27
tobacco industry 14, 21, 23, 27